Overweight People Can Surf

A Health, Fitness, and Nutrition Adventure

By Mark Kaplan

A post pandemic guide for getting to fitness or back to health. The steps and execution for weights, aerobics, nutrition, and surfing.

Other Books:

Creating Your Own Happiness*

The Good Life Plan*

The Surfers Life*

Surf Instructions: Beginner to Advanced*

The Surfing Guide

The Surf Course: 30 page audio book

*Available on Amazon

Table of Contents

Prologue

I have been a surf instructor for 11 years. I am also a Certified Health Coach and have been through Personal Trainer and Nutrition Programs. I have treated surfing and fitness separately even though they are interchangeable and co-dependent. Professional surfers spend more time out of the water training than in the water.

There is a correlation between fitness and the ability to learn to surf, fitness and progressing in surfing. Surfing is one of the more demanding full body sports. It requires strength, flexibility, and stamina. For people who want to learn to surf it often points out the need for conditioning. For people who want to get in shape, surfing is a great goal.

Intro

I have been overwhelmed this surf season by the number of overweight people taking surf lessons. I think it is the pandemic effect. In the past, I would teach a few people over 230 pounds in a season in which I teach over 400 people. This year, I have been getting seemingly one a week.

Being over 230 pounds does not make one obese. The obesity standard established by health professionals is a ratio between height and weight. This will be further defined in the book.

The first question is why are these people taking surf lessons? I think a lot of it is pandemic related since my whole surf business is fluctuating because of pandemic circumstances. It is an outdoor sport at a vacation destination, so people are combining the opportunity to get outdoors and find a recreation. There are so many indoor limitations that have changed lives.

I am also a Certified Health Coach and went through Personal Trainer courses. I, therefore, am interested in people's struggles with weight and conditioning. One of the problems with both improving nutrition and getting in better shape is many entrants consider it an onerous task and almost punishment.

The consequence is that most drop out of health training before the first year is up. Health Coaches and Personal Trainers are schooled on the frequent occurrence of relapse. This is when clients decide everything is too much effort and they were happier suffering with the condition they were experiencing before they became motivated to change.

One of my big surprises is that just about every overweight person who tries surfing says it was a lot of fun even if they couldn't stand up and ride. I was astonished at how they could have fun not achieving what in my mind was the minimum achievement for fun.

Then I realized that in the last 11 years I have been teaching surfing, a lot of people who were not very adept said it was really fun and they often said that soon after being in the water. I was in a sense applying my own standards on what should be fun and make people happy. I thought I was being paid to get people to stand up and ride.

I have also gotten used to just about every student, including those in great shape and with excellent physiques, saying surfing is more difficult than they expected and more tiring than they expected. So, it is safe to say, these two observations are true for most people. Surfing looks easy in the movies. Yet, it is one of the most physical full body sports one can begin.

It would only follow that the more weight a person carried and the less exercise they had engaged in would lead to more difficulties standing and riding on a surfboard. This now applies to everyone from children through seniors. I find that many kids are weak. I suspect it is from too much screen time.

This doesn't mean that it would not be possible for everyone to learn to surf. That is the point of this book. It is also a guide of how to begin a fitness program and progress to great fitness and health. Surfing is fun for most everyone. Getting in shape to surf could be life changing. It may be the focus and goal that would keep people on track to change their lives by becoming healthy. Let's face it, with Covid, there should be extra incentive to remove underlying conditions.

This book will help lead the way to a new lifesytle with the goals of health, self-esteem, fitness, and surfing.

Chapter One

Why Surfers Get Lean

Many people who are beginning to surf can imagine why surfers get lean. It seems apparent to them that the exercise is enough to burn all the fat off one's body. What they don't realize is that a body does get used to a consistent level of exercise. It may require increasing that level to stay lean, but there is more to it than that.

Let's exclude for the moment the fact that so many surfers are teens and are already fat burning machines. Let's look at the post college set and see why they are lean. Not all surfers get to surf every day or often enough to burn everything they eat.

The Phenomena of Being a Surfer

When one begins to fall in love with surfing which for many is the first time they try it, many things can change. There is the thrill of riding a wave. Then there is the connection with the ocean. There becomes a realization that we and the ocean are both parts of Mother Nature together.

A respect develops immediately for the power of the waves and the awesomeness of the water. We become grateful for the opportunity to match our skills with the demands of riding a wave. It usually leads to the desire to ride a bigger one. We start to realize the connection of how being in better physical condition improves our chance and confidence to ride our dream waves.

Getting better at things can create an addiction. Writers, musicians, artists, athletes, chefs, and entrepreneurs develop addictions to their passions because the passions become who they are. We become and identify with what we love. Professional surfers are some of the finest conditioned athletes on earth as they feel the path of surfing better and improving their health as the same path.

If beginner surfers are out of condition but want to be better surfers, it is likely the pursuit will not only increase their spirituality, but their awareness of their physical bodies. Surfing requires strength, flexibility, and stamina. Obviously, good nutrition is necessary to feed the machine. This creates a nice check list of behaviors to develop and maintain.

Chapter Two

Why Is Surfing Such a Great Sport

I first started surfing in high school. There were not as many people surfing as a percentage of the population and few people understood the allure. I bought a 9'6" surfboard which in those days was very heavy. I would drive over the hill to the beach after working the day at my dad's store. I drove to Malibu to ride the famous point break at the Pier.

I was a beginner that had not taken lessons. Most people would have called me a kook because I would get on the wave in front of surfers coming down the wave and block them as I jumped up and fell off. I had no idea of how to surf nor of the existence of surfing etiquette.

I learned by trial and error, but at the end of summer I sold my board and was back in school playing the traditional sports. I didn't get the Nature connection until years later when I would surf on my Hawaii vacations. I started to feel the beauty of being out on a sunny day in warm water and looking down through the clear water and catching a beautiful rolling wave. Aaah, there was something magical about this surfing thing.

I spent my youth going to the beach to enjoy body surfing and riding boogie boards. My main sports other than high school sports of football and swimming were skiing and later snowboarding. I would surf on vacations in Hawaii. It wasn't until I moved to the beach in Oceanside just 12 years ago and began surfing everyday that the magic gripped me.

It frequently grips people right away. They immediately feel the connection to the ocean and Mother Nature. Surfers go out often when there are not good waves just to sit on their boards and enjoy the sun and water. "I'm just going out to get wet", they say.

Some people are intimidated by the ocean. They fear the power and their vulnerability. Even surfers have respect for these two aspects. Surfing becomes an act of managing fear. In lessons, I love to see people get comfortable in the water.

A second fear students often have is of standing up on the surfboard. They fear they are going to fall. Falling is part of the sport, but if you don't stand up, you won't ride. I tell them that fear is the 800 pound gorilla in surfing. Surfers learn to laugh at most falls or they would not go back in the water.

One of my goals is to get people comfortable in the ocean. Once students have learned to ride waves to the beach, I start them paddling out through waves to catch foam waves coming in. This is when the magic often begins for them. Now it is just them and the ocean where they are using their judgement on which waves to allow pass and which ones to catch.

At this point, they will be forever aligned and sympathetic to the ocean and the fun of mingling with its power. Riding a surfboard that has no power and using it to get into something with power is a feeling that is hard to express. It would be like jumping on a skateboard with a sail to catch the wind. Once you experience it, you know exactly what it is.

Chapter Three

The Physical Demands of Surfing

Many people say after surfing lessons "now I know why surfers are so skinny." Being skinny is not a requirement. It could be a worthwhile goal. Surfing a lot could reduce your weight, but consider that a lot of surfers are teenagers and their high metabolism along with the incredible exercise keeps them lean.

It is difficult to exercise off weight without good nutrition. I am now reading a book about hiking the Appalachian Trail. The author says in three weeks he lost 15 pounds off a 157 pound frame that he already thought was lean. There are exceptions on how to lose weight if you want to go to extremes.

In my late 20's, when I was running with the Santa Monica Track Club, I had already been running 5 miles a day 5 days a week and was at my high school graduation weight of 175 pounds. Once I started their routine of running 60 miles a week, I was soon at 165 pounds and people said I looked too skinny. Extreme exercise will shed pounds.

In my 30's while working full time and raising a family, I had put on weight and had blossomed to 225 pounds. When I set a goal of losing 50 pounds, I was already exercising at the gym and hiking most days. It occurred to me that exercise was not enough. I had to change my nutrition. As I started to lose weight and dropped to 200 pounds, my interest in more exercise increased and I increased the intensity. Intensity sheds pounds very fast, but you need to be in shape before adding intensity.

Surfing is intense. It is like doing intervals. The paddling is most of the work. Once the energy stores have been used up paddling, the surf session is not productive. Building muscle through exercise creates greater energy stores in the muscles, so exercisers have more stamina. People who paddle often can paddle longer. People who exercise with weights can paddle easier.

Surfing requires strength in a ratio to the surfer's weight. I have noticed these days that kids tend to be weak. Too much screen time. There is no longer the interest in running around outdoors and playing with their friends climbing trees, riding bikes, and getting on jungle gyms.

Too many jobs are sedentary and the first thing that occurs is a lack of flexibility. Flexibility includes the hamstrings, buttocks, and lower back. A burpee exercises all three. Squats are great and so are dead lifts. Yoga of course is ideal and so is gymnastics.

A surfer should easily touch his palms to the floor without bending his knees. Experienced surfers and professionals stretch to minimize injury and create the smooth flow necessary. Start stretching slowly and it is best to engage after a walk or other exercise. It is great to be able to move freely and pick things up without worrying about back problems.

Stamina is built slowly. In personal training we start sedentary people with walking. Then as time passes, we move to longer and more frequent walks. At a certain point people can start running. The same process begins with running. Start slow and eventually add intensity. If you are sedentary, give yourself a year to have an intense running program.

Other aerobic exercises like swimming, biking and treadmills can be gentle introductions to aerobics and allow the addition of intervals for intensity. As a person progresses in these areas, they will notice their proficiency at surfing improves. They start to see the possibilities.

Chapter Four

What is Overweight or Obesity?

There is a health care definition of body size which is a ratio between height and weight. The result is called the Body Mass Index (BMI). It has its shortfalls like in measuring people that are heavily muscled or have heavy bones and possibly calling them overweight when it isn't true. Other than a few exceptions, the Index satisfies most people in the medical fields.

People can say the Index is not a true measure. Over the last 50+ years most people in the health care and medical industry are comfortable with the measurements. If it is in error for your particular case, it is not in error by much.

The BMI is calculated by dividing your weight in centimeters by your height in kilograms.*

For instance, a person is 5'9" and weighs 214 pounds.

His height in meters is calculated by converting it to inches and multiplying by .0254.   5'9" converted to inches is 69 inches multiplied by 0254 is 1.753 meters

His weight at 214 pounds is divided by 2.2 to convert to kilograms to pounds which is 97.3 kg.

The BMI is equal to 97.3 divided by 1.753 (squared) then divided by 100 which equals 31.7 kg/m. You can Google to find your BMI in a chart.

The BMI chart has measures for people that are lean and super fit which differ for men and women. We are more concerned in this book with weights from normal to obesity. Less than 18 on the BMI scale is considered underweight. People extremely fit may be less than 18 as well as people with eating disorders.

18 to 24.9 is considered normal weight. 25 to 29.9 is considered overweight. 30 to 39.9 is considered obese. Over 40 is considered morbid obesity or extreme obesity.

The upper limits of normal are:

5'2" and 136 pounds

6' and 184 pounds

Some examples of obese are:

5'2" and 164 pounds

6' and 221 pounds

Some examples of extremely obese are:

5'2" and 218 pounds

6' and 294 pounds

*Data supplied by Ace Fitness

Health coaches and personal trainers can work with obese people but reach restrictions with extremely obese. These categories require a doctor's clearance. Health professionals start with checking blood pressure and pulse rates. They want doctors' clearance to be sure there are no underlying conditions like diabetes, cardiovascular disease, or any other complications before beginning exertion.

Anyone that is obese or extremely obese should be sure to get medical clearance before initiating physical exercise regimens. Personal trainers would begin these clients with some agility tests, then exercises without weights and encourage walking 10 to 15 minutes a day.

All recommendations in this book will assume the readers have obtained medical clearance before beginning exercises. Nutrition is also an issue. Regular dieting may not be sufficient. Working with programs designed for weight loss may be advisable. At some points, weight loss has to be executed with medical supervision so as not to endanger the client.

In extreme cases, surgery may be recommended to the stomach to restrict food absorption. Many people may first have to work on weight control before beginning exercise. Exercise places a strain on all systems and could result in heart attacks or strokes.

Chapter Five

Easy Diet Considerations

One weight loss organization that counsels personal trainers has a kind and effective way of beginning with overweight and obese clients. They have found that their process results in clients staying on a fitness and nutrition program for up to 5 years as opposed to a great number of people who work with personal trainers and nutritionists only conforming for a year. Old habits die hard.

In the mentioned organization's philosophy, they begin without discussing diet or exercise. They want people to build awareness first. Chances are people that are overweight or obese have already tried a number of times to get fit or lose weight and found the process uncomfortable or unattainable.

Awareness comes from asking some questions. Questions will be like:

Do you eat only things you like or will you also eat things you don't like?

Do you eat when you are not hungry?

Do you know when you are full and then stop?

Do you have emotional triggers that cause you to reach for food?

Do you eat when you are bored?

These are good beginning questions that people should consider each day when entertaining a program to lose weight and get fit. The first step is to realize what and why they eat.

At any point a nutritionist or health coach can help you classify the foods you typically eat and ask you to keep records so that in a week's time you have a good idea of what you are eating and the amount of calories you consume. The most obvious process for losing weight is to burn more calories than are consumed. After a diet is implemented, an exercise program begins to accelerate the number of calories burned.

There are formulas to be discussed in Chapter 15 that will begin to match the average amount of activity you experience a day with the amount of calories you should consume to maintain weight or lose weight. A sedentary person should consume fewer calories than an active person.

Matching consumption with activity becomes the program for losing weight and getting fit. As activity increases, a person can consume more calories. It is important that these are the right calories and that is where the test comes for many people.

There are foods that are considered empty calories or calories that will lead to gaining weight. Foods can be inflammatory for individuals. The foods that are desirable are healthy foods that deliver calories and will contribute to health and weight loss.

Often weight gain is caused by food addictions. Drinking sodas all day may be an addiction. Eating fast food loaded with grease, salt, and fat could be an addiction. Desserts and candy can be addictions.

When I began my 50-pound weight loss, I was addicted to having ice cream every night after dinner. I decided to start there. I found a great trick that has served me ever since. I would jump to something that was possibly also bad but broke the ice cream habit. My choice was Snickers bars. After a week, when the ice cream addiction was broken, I jumped to granola bars.

Then with each food I eliminated, I added one food that was good for me. We know that the recommended foods are mainly fruits and vegetables. Nuts, seeds, and good fats are also recommended but that comes later.

In a slow process of eliminating bad foods and adding good foods, I converted my daily intake. It wasn't long before my 225 pounds was 215 pounds and then 200 pounds. I did it in a slow process so that I could easily adapt and I was not torturing myself or creating cravings.

I was already an exerciser, but as I lost weight, I could more easily increase my exercise and the intensity. Once again, the idea is to possibly wait for the exercise program until the nutrition program is showing signs of progress.

As I progressed, the foods dropping off my consumption list were sugar, flour, bad fats, and most restaurant foods. This selection starts eliminating bad snacks, desserts, bread, pasta, and sodas. You might already imagine what would happen to your weight if you eliminated these items.

Then you learn to consume what is remaining which include fruits, vegetables, lean meats, nuts, seeds, and good fats. At the end of the 4 years, I had progressed to a raw diet where I didn't cook anything and therefore was not eating meats other than canned tuna. I only ate very natural foods. The weight was dropping off so fast in combination with intense exercise that I stopped the raw diet and began to eat a more complete diet.

One of the best diet plans I have found is in the book "The Plan" by Lyn Genet-Recitas. She has tested her plan on 1,000's of patients and determined the foods with the least inflammatory properties. One starts the first three days with some of these foods and then begins adding a new food each day.

The truth is the inflammation of foods creates the weight gain. On her plan, a person should lose a half pound a day. If you stay the same or gain weight, something you ate was inflammatory. The next caveat is you have to consume a lot of water. You need to drink 8 to 10 glasses a day but there are formulas for how much water to drink according to your weight.

The body will use food to extract water, if necessary, so the secret is staying hydrated so the body can digest the food properly. I still find the secret to maintaining weight is drinking a lot of water. It takes a while to build the ability to drink water and create thirst.

There is a great book on water called "Your Body's Many Cries for Water" by F. Batmanghelidj, M.D. It will emphasize the importance of water in our bodies. After all, we are about 70% water and a bunch of minerals.

Chapter Six

Catching Waves

The fun of surfing for beginners starts with catching waves. Many students who don't learn to stand up say they had great fun. Laying on a surfboard and feeling a foam wave start to push the board at 15 mph is exhilarating. Standing, of course, would be more fun, but just the feeling of being pushed by pure energy is a great reward. Waves are water energized by the wind.

Catching waves becomes the obsession of surfers for the rest of their lives. The better they become, the bigger waves they could ride. The second aspect is recognizing waves and how to catch them. Waves from day to day, low tide to high tide, and beach to beach are different.

The beginner surfer first learns how to roll over onto a surfboard as the foam wave is approaching and begins paddling to start the momentum. The surfer then looks back to see how close the foam wave is to the board. When the wave is only a few feet away, he paddles much harder in order to get in front of the wave.

The surfer does not want to remain with the tail of the surfboard in the foam as he tries to stand up. He wants to accelerate so the surfboard is being pushed by the little curved lip that is created as the foam waves moves to shore. This is where the smooth pop up and ride exist.

After the surfer learns how to catch the foam waves and ride to the beach, he can progress by paddling out through the waves and turning around to catch the next one. This begins to help surfers get comfortable in the ocean as they start selecting which waves to ride.

Paddling longer builds stamina quicker. Paddling is what makes surfers tired. This is the game. Paddle more to build stamina. It is like running. Start with a quarter mile and build stamina until you can run a mile.

Correct paddling occurs by dropping the arm into the water up to the elbow so most of the power is generated by the forearm. Strokes should be short and close to the board. Surfers do not want to hand paddle. Strokes should also be even with both arms. Many have a tendency when they begin in foam waves to paddle harder with one arm causing the board to carve sideways into the wave and then get turned over.

A high-volume surfboard makes paddling easier but not necessarily easy. There is still lots of work involved. If a person wanted to make paddling their exercise program, they could burn a lot of calories, build muscle, gain balance on the surfboard, get more comfortable in the ocean and improve a basic surfing skill.

Chapter Seven

Ways to Build Upper Body and Core Strength

Surfing is a full body sport. It begins with paddling. Paddling builds the arms, back, and shoulders. Surfing requires going from laying down on the surfboard to a standing position while moving through the water on a board that can sink from a person's body weight while moving. This requires upper body, lower body, and core strength. The smaller or lower volume the surfboard, the more it sinks.

Naturally, surfing would build the requisite strength with consistent engagement. Most professional athletes spend more time out of the water building these strengths than they spend in the water. One way to improve one's level of proficiency in the water is to also train out of the water.

Stamina and flexibility are also important and will be treated in the next chapters. One can see that surfing looks so easy in the movies, but viewers have no idea how much training, practice, and time were spent on the skills to make it look easy. In fact, very few people who learn think it is easy.

This is why I am amazed at how many people that are out of shape want to learn to surf, but happy they do and see it as an opportunity to improve their lives. There is this allusion created by film that anyone can do it. I am happy to say that 95% of my students are riding in the first lesson. I am sad to say that people who are too overweight, not flexible, or too weak to lift their bodies off the surfboard have a lot of trouble.

The idea of this book is to help overweight, obese, and people out of condition get into shape so they can stand up on a surfboard and enjoy what others are enjoying. It might be a good goal that gets one through the unpleasant discipline of doing things that are new and not as satisfying or maybe even torture compared to existing routines.

My favorite exercises for building all these necessary body strengths are just a few. I love squats, dead lifts, burpies, cable pulls, bench presses and pushups. These exercises work the biggest muscle groups and build flexibility at the same time. I will mention them throughout the book.

A personal trainer will first test a person for agility and the ability to maintain balance doing a few things like squats or perhaps lunges. Then he will create a variety of exercises without weights. After a person has demonstrated competence in these beginning exercises, he will begin to introduce light weights.

A person can learn exercise routines on YouTube. There are videos on the proper form for each exercise. Proper form prevents injury especially important for squats and dead lifts. These exercises could be performed at home during a time when Covid makes gym attendance undesirable.

Chapter Eight

The Desirability of Building Muscle

There are five very good reasons for building muscle:

- Muscle begins to absorb the glucose created by carbohydrates instead of letting them pass directly to fat.
- Muscle builds energy reserves that allow you to exercise longer.
- Muscle building allows the body to execute more demanding feats.
- Muscle will burn fat to recover.
- Muscle will burn fat for fuel.

Surfing requires muscle. These days kids often lack muscle because they have become so adapted to the screen life and spend little time outdoors running and climbing or even throwing a ball. Muscle can be built from a number of fun activities that don't have to be training.

Swimming, riding a bike, and hiking are all excellent for muscle building and aerobics. More formal activities might include a treadmill, pulling cables, and lifting weights. You want to be sure to check with your doctor to see that activities you have not engaged in to this point are acceptable for your conditioning and health.

Professional counselors including personal trainers, clinics, or doctors might suggest you lose weight first and start off with more walking to build your heart and cardiovascular system.

The Psychological Advantages of Building Fitness

There are several good reasons to get fit:

- Self-esteem
- Gain respect
- Better job opportunities
- Better lifestyle
- Look better in clothes
- Mating opportunities

- Better health
- More activities
- More energy
- Disease immunity
- Longer life

One of the great results of starting a program and achieving some progress is you get more encouraged as you progress. One of the most important characteristics you could develop is discipline. Discipline opens up an entire world of what you can accomplish.

You will find that getting in shape is just the beginning once you develop discipline. Once you realize you have the ability to set a goal and stick to the work, you start to think could achieve anything. All those dreams that require you to set a goal and work towards that goal become achievable.

Progress comes one step at a time. There are few naturals at anything. Most accomplished athletes, artists, musicians, and business people had to put in the work one day at a time. What they have learned is that progress comes with focus and practice. Humans have evolved applying just these processes. If you want to be different, you just have to focus and practice with discipline. There is plenty of support available in the world for your efforts.

Chapter Nine

Ways to Build Stamina

Building stamina can be fun and rewarding because you can realize progress and it can be measured. It is easy to know that at the beginning you could only walk for ten minutes and then you are walking for 30 minutes. Then you are running a mile. Then you are running five miles.

Personal trainers have established four categories for aerobic exercise. The first is exercise that barely raises your heart-beat and in which you could exercise and talk comfortably. This might include walking or a treadmill.

The second level includes a little more intensity by increasing the duration the frequency or the speed. It makes exercising and talking a little more difficult. It will also include adding some intensity in some sort of interval process. The intervals can be very short. The advantage of intervals is they speed up the heart, build cardiovascular, and improve fat burning.

The third level will include intensity training that comes closer to your maximum capacity. At this point, exercising and talking will be difficult. It will still be mostly low-level intensity on a weekly basis but will introduce more intensity as duration, speed, and frequency.

The fourth level is for athletes who compete. They may have the need to perform at maximum capacity in their event or at the end when there is a sprint to win. They practice closer to maximum capacity. They still spend most of their time at a low-level aerobic level to build capacity and only test their maximum perhaps once a week.

A person could train and run a 10K operating in just the second level. A person who wanted to run half or full marathons would be in level three. Increasing duration with occasional intervals develops the capacity for most people to engage in the activities they enjoy. The more serious minded can move to higher levels of aerobic activity because they want to maximize their fitness or they have other specific goal(s).

Maybe one person wants to run a 10K and another wants to climb Mount Everest. We can pick our own goals and engage in the practices we enjoy or think are appropriate.

Chapter Ten

Ways to Build Flexibility

These days people have lost flexibility from so many sedentary behaviors. We have been locked down for over a year. Now many are starting to enjoy their remote work and schooling. During the process, many previous activities have been closed and it may take people a while to reengage.

Sedentary behavior tightens our hamstrings, buttocks, and lower back. All three need to be loosened for surfing. They also should be loose to make all activities both more enjoyable and injury free.

There are a lot of activities that are easier if there is flexibility. Just picking things up off the floor requires flexibility. Flexibility prevents injury from lifting boxes or moving in unusual ways. People who are very active can also lose flexibility. Runners and triathletes who don't stretch can have very tight hamstrings and lower backs.

Flexibility is key to surfing because a person lying on the surfboard has to push up their chest and place their back foot under their butt flat on the board. Not everyone can do this. The next step is to stand on that foot and raise the hands while moving the other foot to the front of the board.

These moves utilize upper body strength, leg strength, and core strength. All these abilities could be built from yoga or gymnastics. A few weight activities are very helpful. I like squats, dead lifts, and burpies to build flexibility and strength. Add pushups and the package for surfing is pretty complete.

At the beginning, try to touch the floor with your fingers. You might find that you have a long way to go. Stretching to affect your flexibility takes time. You want to be careful because too much of a strain can cause a muscle pull.

An easy to perform stretch is pushing against a wall with one leg bent for support and the other leg stretched to exercise the calf.

Sitting on the ground with legs spread and leaning forward will introduce you to the tightness of your hamstrings.

There are a variety of floor exercises to stretch the hamstrings and lower back. It may take time before you can attempt them. Once you can, they are a good path for daily growth in flexibility. It can take a month before you see progress in stretching. Be patient and don't overstretch and pull something.

At a point you might be able to lift one leg and hold your toes. This is one of the best exercises for stretching your buttocks. People don't think of their buttocks as needing stretching, but physical therapists and counselors in rehab will stress that our buttocks need to be stretched.

Gaining flexibility in our calves, hamstrings, buttocks, and lower back open up opportunities for enjoying more activities and recreation. It is great to engage in a new activity and not have to worry about injury.

Chapter Eleven

Standing up On the Surfboard

Standing up on the surfboard is a main objective in surfing. Two others are catching waves and then riding them. The process of catching waves and standing up is about timing and rhythm.

Whether foam waves or real waves, the surfer sees the wave and makes a judgement about position and timing. As a beginner, you see foam waves arriving and decide when to roll over to start paddling and catch the wave.

In catching the foam wave, the surfer begins by rolling over 20 feet before the wave arrives noticing how big, how fast, and if it is coming at an angle. Then he starts paddling to get some momentum. As the wave gets close, the surfer paddles hard as the wave hits the board and until he feels the surfboard take off in front of the wave.

Then the surfer places his hands on the surfboard next to his chest in a man's push up position. Then he pushes and places his back foot on the surfboard flat and under his butt. The foot placement is about two feet from the tail and in the middle of the surfboard. The surfer stands on the rear foot/leg as he brings up his hands and moves the other foot close to the nose of the board.

When standing in the correct posture, the front and rear foot need to be about shoulder width apart and the front foot has to be close enough to the nose to hold it down but not so close the foot pushes the nose under water.

The correct posture on the surfboard is with the weight equal on the front and rear leg with the torso upright. The hips and shoulders are square to the front and the hands in front where they can be seen. If the posture is correct, the surfboard will go straight and little work or balance is needed.

People think surfing is about balance, but I have seen very few people who did not have adequate balance. The downfall is not executing the pop up properly and smoothly to arrive in the right posture. If the weight is not distributed correctly by having the weight equal on the right and left sides of the middle stringer of the surfboard, balance will not help much.

I have students practice this pop up on their living room floor. If you want to test your mettle, try it in your living room. It might be a window into your ability and the work you have to do to get in surf shape.

Chapter Twelve

A Good Beginning Weight Training Program

Weightlifting is known as a good practice to build muscle and get in shape. What is not usually discussed is that it creates receptors for accepting glucose out of the blood stream. Glucose is converted from carbohydrates.

If the muscles are not absorbing glucose, any excess carbohydrate consumption goes to fat. This would include sugar, flour, and even carbohydrates from too many vegetables and fruits. If muscle is not accepting glucose, too much may remain in the blood stream causing high blood sugar.

An overweight person might not like weightlifting. Maybe previous attempts were too difficult or results were not seen. It is a slow process, but one in which progress is usually detectable. They say 5 pounds of new muscle will burn an extra 95,000 calories a year. That would translate to about 30 pounds of body fat.

What is great about a muscle building program is that muscles use fat for fuel and recovery. They also use glucose. Our body will only store a certain amount of glucose and then if it is not used, the remainder is transported to fat for future use. Between the liver, the muscles, and the blood stream, the average body will store about 900 calories of glucose from carbohydrates. This also gives you and idea about how much you should consume at one time. The more intense your physical exercise, the more calories you can consume.

The more muscles are developed, the more glucose they will store and then the more carbohydrates one can eat without gaining weight. A trained athlete knows when to eat and what to eat to complement his efforts.

At the beginning, a personal trainer may not have an overweight or obese person lifting weights. They begin with exercises that require balance and mobility. Exercises such as squats and lunges help the beginner build balance and start to burn some calories.

The beginner exerciser wants lots of repetitions to condition the body. The repetitions build cardiovascular capability, exert little strain on muscles, and minimize the chance of injury. Learning form is important to facilitate this process.

After a few months, a personal trainer might introduce light weights. Maybe five or ten pounds to do some of the floor exercises. Then the exerciser might proceed to machines. The great advantage of machines over dumbbells and barbells, is they control the motion to help maintain form and minimize chances of injury.

In lifting weights for the beginner, a good routine is ten exercises with 25 reps and three sets of each with a light weight. A complete routine should build to an hour or hour and a half. As time progresses, the exerciser can increase weights and intensity.

Increasing intensity could be more weight, more sets, and less rest in between sets. This will begin to build cardiovascular capability, muscle's need for glucose, and stamina. When the muscles run low on glucose they search for fat.

This type of routine could be engaged five days a week with only two days rest. The muscles are not strained and have little need for recovery. An exerciser, at this point, is utilizing only 40% to 60% of their one lift maximum capacity. The maximum capacity is a guess at the beginning.

As exercisers progress into the second level or stage, they begin to do fewer reps with more weight. This utilizes a different type of muscle. You can learn about fast and slow twitch muscles. The exerciser is lifting weights between 60% and 80% of one lift maximum capacity with 12 to 15 reps and three sets. Building intensity once again comes from doing more weight and more sets. Doing more weights and sets increases the duration of the total exercise session.

At this point, the muscles may need to be rested for recovery. Muscle growth occurs during rest periods in which muscles take on protein and fuel. At this point, an exerciser could probably engage three to four times a week.

The final stage is where real strength and muscle building begin. The exerciser starts utilizing weights that test maximum capacity and doing only five to eight repetitions and three sets. At this stage, the exerciser may be lifting 80% to 95% of capacity. He may only be doing five repetitions and three sets. He may finish with one set at maximum capacity.

This stage requires lots of recovery. At this stage, the exerciser may only engage in this routine once a week and lift lighter a few times a week. Many normal exercisers do not need to reach the third stage. Most goals can be met in level two.

Chapter Thirteen

A Good Beginning Aerobic Program

Building cardiovascular fitness is a long-term process that requires patience, consistency, discipline, focus, willpower, and goals. It has to start with the first step.

Running a marathon could be a long-term goal. It could start with walking which leads to running. A person starts with a few minutes a day and increases intensity by adding duration. A beginning of 10 minutes a day can lead to 30 minutes a day and 150 minutes a week. Soon the program builds to an hour a day and therefore five hours a week.

A friend of mine wanted to climb to the base camp of Mount Everest at 17,500 feet. He was not in great condition. He started walking four miles and built it to twenty miles. He stretched and did weight training over a year's period- of-time. He made it.

As a teenager I enjoyed jogging when no one else was engaged. It did become a national craze. I started with a mile at my high school track. Then in college I was running three miles. As an adult I started running four miles a day five days a week along a great grass strip in my town. A friend introduced me to a track club and before long I was running sixty miles a week.

At first aerobics might seem a struggle. It might require great will power and determination that develops into discipline. Discipline is one of the greatest characteristics we can develop for success. One realizes that if you can stick to a plan, anything is achievable.

As a health coach and personal trainer, I would suggest to someone that they begin walking 10 to 15 minutes a day and slowly build the duration and the frequency. These are two characteristics of progress; duration and frequency. They apply to all the aerobic exercises. The third characteristic could be intensity which in running is speed or shorter rest time between intervals. Intervals are considered the fastest way to achieve progress in aerobics.

As beginning exercisers start with walking and increase duration and frequency, they might become runners. As runners progress with duration and frequency, they might then introduce intervals. As intervals are introduced, a person's speed keeps increasing. As club runners, we frequently engaged in workouts of running intervals to increase our average running speed.

At this point the exerciser may desire competition. Simple competitions might be 3K and 6K runs which are approximately 3 and 6 miles. The next step is half marathons and then maybe marathons which are 13 miles and 26 miles. They, of course, can be runs for just personal best times and are not necessarily pitted against other runners except at a very high level.

People who really love exercise and want to test themselves get into endurance activities like triathlons or long bike rides. RAAM is Race Across America in a bike ride that starts in Oceanside, CA and ends in Maryland, 3,000 miles away. Consider the duress of riding a bike 22 hours a day for 8 days.

Duration runners also do ultra-marathons of 50 and 100 miles. Then if that is not enough, they introduce tough terrain by running in the mountains or running across scorching deserts.

On the other hand, consider what the human body can do and how far most of us are from reaching our potential. Why does an ultra-athlete engage in such strenuous activity? It starts slowly. They find that they enjoy and are good at a certain activity. As they build stamina, they are always wondering how much more they could do. That's how it starts. One middle aged man who was riding long distance bike races said he discovered he had the aptitude.

Whereas exercise may start as a chore, it can soon become the center of your life. Runners are runners and surfers are surfers, and mountain climbers or hikers are the same. People start identifying themselves with their passion classifying themselves first with that passion and saying that is who I am and why I am here.

With each type of recreation, there are usually activities that enhance performance in that activity. Surfing is a great recreation but benefits from building strength and stamina outside the actual surfing time. Professionals probably spend more time cross training than surfing. Mountain climbers spend a lot of time climbing smaller mountains before they climb the big ones. Preparing to surf might start by walking ten minutes a day.

Chapter Fourteen

A Good Beginning Nutrition Program

Losing and maintaining weight is a long-term mission. Most people who want to lose ten pounds in a month put it back on if they were successful in losing the weight. As I mentioned earlier, a good organization that works with Health Coaches in training overweight people suggests that exercise and diet should not be mentioned at the beginning.

The first steps include becoming aware of eating habits. The second would be to start cleaning out the cupboards and refrigerator of items that should not be eaten. Third would be to start analyzing what is eaten on a typical day and during a typical week. Nutritionists and health coaches may supply a list of foods and ask the client to check which ones are normally consumed, the quantity, and the frequency.

Once the coach and client are aware of what is consumed and determine the probable amount of calories and the balance between protein, carbohydrates, and fat, the coach or nutritionist will make suggestions.

Overweight and obese people may need to be supervised by a doctor or work with a professional clinic or weight loss commercial program. Sometimes surgery is recommended to tie off the stomach and reduce intake.

For people that are overweight, a health coach or trainer will start them on a combination of nutrition and exercise programs. Losing weight is mathematics. We know that you have to burn more calories than you consume. In weight training, it is possible to not lose weight but lose fat and inches. Muscle is heavier than fat.

A pound is approximately 3300 calories. Reducing the amount of calories consumed by 500 calories over the amount burned a day will reduce weight by a pound in a week. There are charts to determine approximately how many calories a person might burn in a day depending upon the level of their physical activity. One is shown in Chapter 15.

The more calories a person burns, the more calories they can consume. A very active athlete does not want to lose weight, so they need to consume a large amount of the proper calories. A sedentary person needs less.

One issue is a person's metabolism. A sedentary person has a low rate of metabolism and doesn't burn many calories while at rest. The idea of exercise is to increase the rate of metabolism to burn more calories while at rest.

A second issue is that people can't starve to lose weight. Starving slows down the metabolism because the body fears the person is really starving and it wants to preserve fat stores. It is usually better to reduce calories and eat enough so the body does not think it is being starved. Early man did starve in the winters and the body slowed his metabolism to keep him alive.

Fasting for periods of time can be useful. Many weightlifters who want to lose fat while gaining muscle eat in shortened time periods or windows to allow the body more time to digest and burn fuel. They may eat within an 8-hour window or 6-hour window. This gives the body a lot of time to burn fuel.

When I lost 50 pounds over a 4-year period, I slowly began to remove bad calories and substitute with good calories such as fruits and vegetables. After a while the body doesn't crave the bad foods and the mind even puts up resistance when you think you want something bad.

At the beginning, the mind will sabotage all your good efforts. This becomes a battle of who is in control. You have to act as an observer of what the mind is telling you and fight against the mind if the food doesn't align with your goals. As the mind sees progress, it becomes your best supporter.

Chapter Fifteen

Calculating Calories Burned a Day

It is important in losing weight to first determine how many calories are being consumed a day. Then calculate approximately how many calories are being burned. Weight gain and loss are the differences between these two. It's that simple most of the time unless there are genetic or underlying conditions.

This article from https://medicalnewstoday.com explains how to calculate the number of calories a person burns a day depending on several factors.

"The Harris-Benedict formula is a relatively simple process in which a person multiplies their basal metabolic rate (BMR) by their average daily activity level.

BMR is the number of calories a person burns by simply existing. BMR varies based on age, sex, size, and genetics. To calculate BMR, a person uses inches for height, pounds for weight, and years for age in the following formulas:

- **For men**: 66 + (6.2 x weight) + (12.7 x height) – (6.76 x age)

- **For women**: 655.1 + (4.35 x weight) + (4.7 x height) – (4.7 x age)

The results of the BMR calculation are then used to multiply against the average daily activity of the person. Points are awarded based on how active a person is.

Points for activity levels are as follows:

- 1.2 points for a person who does little to no exercise

- 1.37 points for a slightly active person who does light exercise 1–3 days a week

- 1.55 points for a moderately active person who performs moderate exercise 3–5 days a week

- 1.725 points for a very active person who exercises hard 6–7 days a week

- 1.9 points for an extra active person who either has a physically demanding job or has a particularly challenging exercise routine.

When the BMR is calculated and the activities points are determined, the two scores are multiplied. The total is the number of calories burned on an average day.

For example, to calculate how many calories a 37-year-old, 6-foot-tall, and 170-pound man who is moderately active burns, the formula would look like:

$$(66 + (6.2 \times 170) + (12.7 \times 72) - (6.76 \times 37)) \times 1.55 = 2{,}663$$
$$\text{calories/day}$$

This figure shows that a man of this age, height, weight, and activity level can consume 2,663 calories and maintain his current weight. He could increase or decrease weight by consuming more or less than this amount over the course of several days.

For those who do not wish to make the calculations themselves, there are a range of calorie calculators available online. Most use a similar formula to work out calories burned.

A doctor or nutritionist should also be able to help people work out how many calories they burn each day.

Factors affecting calorie burn:

Many factors affect how many calories a person burns each day. Some of the factors that influence daily calorie burn are not in a person's control while others can be changed.

These factors include:

- **Age**: the older a person is, the fewer calories burned per day.
- **Sex**: men burn more calories than women.
- **Amount of daily activity**: those who move more, burn more calories.
- **Body composition**: those with more muscle burn more calories than those who have less muscle.

- **Body size**: larger people burn more calories than smaller people, even at rest.

- **Thermogenesis**: this is the amount of energy the body uses to break down food.

- **Pregnancy**: pregnant women burn more calories than non-pregnant women.

- **Breast-feeding**: women who are breast-feeding also burn extra calories.

Calories burned by exercise or activities

All activities use up calories, even housework such as vacuuming. More intense physical activity such as aerobics will burn more calories.

Calorie counts for exercise and activity will vary from person to person. Age, sex, body type, and size influence how many calories an individual will burn doing a physical activity.

In general, more intense or strenuous activity will burn more calories than lighter effort exercise.

The following calorie counts are based on a 155-pound person doing the following exercise or activity for 30 minutes:

- aerobics: 211

- stationary bike (light effort): 176
- stationary bike (moderate effort): 247
- dusting: 70
- gardening: 176
- grocery shopping: 106
- hiking: 211
- house cleaning: 106
- jogging: 247
- running 12-minute miles: 282
- running 10-minute miles: 352
- running 7.5-minute miles: 428
- laundry, including folding clothes: 70
- mowing the lawn (no riding mowers): 141
- playing with kids at the playground: 141
- cooking: 70
- raking: 141
- shoveling snow: 211
- tennis (singles): 282
- vacuuming: 70
- brisk walking: 141
- walking while pushing a stroller: 70

- weightlifting: 106

- yoga: 141

Anyone that wants to figure out how many calories they burn can input their statistics into a calorie calculator and find personalized results.

Weight-loss tips

People looking to lose weight should try to create a calorie deficit by following these tips:

- moving more

- eating a lower calorie diet full of healthful fruits, vegetables, and lean proteins

- getting enough sleep

- drinking more water

Losing weight can be very tough to do. Understanding how many calories an individual's body burns per day and what to do to increase daily calorie burn is the key to success."

Chapter Sixteen

Learning to Stand Up on the Surfboard

Surfing requires upper body strength, leg strength, core strength, and stamina. People that put-on weight are often not exercising. In learning to surf, this is more of a problem than weight because there are lots of overweight surfers.

Surfing is a lot easier if a surfer is lean. There is the power to weight ratio which means the power to lift one's body off the surfboard. This would mean that regardless of the weight, if a surfer is strong enough, they can get their body into a standing position on the surfboard. I recently has a strong surfing student who was 260 pounds and did a nice job of riding the surfboard.

The upper body pushes the body off the surfboard to begin the pop up. But upper body strength is also needed to paddle. When a surfer gets tired paddling, the fatigue seeps through their body and they begin to falter in all areas.

Leg strength is needed to stand up on the surfboard. In the beginner pop up, the surfer has to stand up on their rear leg. This means that while in a lying down position, the surfer puts their rear foot on the board and lifts their entire weight up as they move the other foot to the front of the surfboard.

This is where flexibility is also crucial. The rear foot when placed on the surfboard must be placed under the butt and flat on the board. If a person is not well stretched, they cannot get their foot flat. If their foot is not flat, they cannot stand on it. Try touching the floor without bending your knees. This is a first indication of your flexibility. Putting your palms on the floor is better.

As mentioned earlier, flexibility is needed in the hamstrings, buttocks, and lower back. All three get tight in sedentary behavior. When a person is capable of exercise, the best two exercises for loosening these three areas are burpies and squats. Both can be engaged without weights. The burpies require cardiovascular fitness, so be careful.

Upper body strength is developed with pushups, bench presses, and cable pulls. They work together to give the strength to push off the surfboard and to paddle. Of course, nothing works for paddling like getting in the ocean and paddling or swimming. Swimming can be enjoyed anywhere without the need for the ocean and it is great cardiovascular training.

The process of standing up on the surfboard begins with catching the wave. Then the surfer places his hands on the surfboard in a man's push up position next to the chest. The surfer pushes up and puts their rear (right foot for most people) on the surfboard flat. Flat is crucial. The foot is slightly turned to the right. When the front foot lands, it will also be turned at a 45 degree angle to the right.

Then the surfer stands on that rear foot, and raises his hands and body as he moves the other foot to the nose of the board. The finishing stance should have the feet about shoulder width apart (3'). The hips and shoulders should be square to the front with both hands in front. Knees are flexed and weight is equal on front and back legs.

At this point the surfer is riding balanced to the beach. If the posture is correct, the surfboard will travel straight with very little work required to stay on the surfboard. If the posture is not correct, the surfer struggles to stay on the surfboard.

Chapter Seventeen

Selecting the Right Surfboard

Beginners want to select a surfboard with a lot of volume to make learning to surf easier and also allow them to advance until such a time they may want to surf a shorter soft top board or purchase a hard board. Volume is calculated by multiplying length, times width, times thickness. There is a chart at the end of the book that matches weight with the volume of surfboard that should be purchased.

Beginners should start with high volume boards and move slowly in buying boards with less volume. Surfing progress is usually slow and moving to an advanced board can lead to more frustration than fun.

A beginner wants more volume for four reasons. They are easier to paddle. They catch foam waves easier. They are easier for doing the pop up. They are easier to ride. If any one of these gets more difficult, the fun drains out of the experience.

The beginner surfer begins near the shore rolling over onto the surfboard to catch foam waves and rides to the beach. The surfer then progresses to paddling out to ride bigger foam waves and starts catching small real waves. The soft top high-volume surfboard is great for this practice. The surfer should keep progressing trying to catch bigger real waves.

At this point, the beginner is now an intermediate surfer. On real waves, he will learn to drop down a small face. Then he will learn to angle the surfboard toward the pocket to prevent pearling (where the nose goes under water) before popping up. He may also learn bottom turns, cut- backs, and accelerating.

Now, he may decide he would like a hard board to improve maneuverability. The main advantage of a hard board over a soft top is that the rails are thinner to allow the surfer to dig the rail into the wave for sharper carves. Up to this point, there is no need to jump to a hard board.

The progress to shorter hard boards from soft tops should be very gradual. The surfer should buy boards just 6 inches shorter at a time trying to maintain good width and thickness. As soon as the volume drops, the paddling is more difficult, catching waves requires more advanced timing, popping up is more unstable, and riding is more unstable.

One way to progress is to move to lower volume soft tops. I often start surfers on a 9' soft top and move them to an 8' soft top. An 8' soft top is a great board and could last a surfer all their life, especially if they don't get in the ocean often. I still ride an 8' soft top and lots of surfers in the line up are riding them. You can ride 7' high waves with them. I also have short boards.

Overweight surfers want at least a 9-foot soft top surfboard. Surfers over 200 pounds would be better served by soft tops that are at least 24 inches wide and near three inches thick. This should suffice up to about 260 pounds. After that, a beginner should consider Stand Up Paddle (SUP) boards. A 9'6" SUP can be 33 inches wide and over 4 inches thick.

Start with the appropriate high-volume surfboard as you begin to lose weight. As a surfer loses weight, they can consider progressing to lower volume soft tops. There are also high-volume hard boards. Hard boards are available up to 12 feet long and have big widths and thickness.

I think a good-sized hard board if a surfer doesn't want to go shorter are boards that are 9' or 9'6". Width and thickness can be varied for better flotation. These boards have lots of volume and are still maneuverable. Lots of surfers are on these boards and the long board surfer has a certain style that usually has them gathering together on beaches where the waves favor long boards. This is usually a reef where the waves form slowly and have nice shape. Sand bar bottom beaches don't allow the waves to form as slowly and often have what are called "close out" waves. These waves are steep and can cause long boards to pearl more easily.

Chapter Eighteen

Selecting a Wetsuit

Wetsuits make surfing comfortable when the water is colder than you personally would enjoy in your swim trunks. Everyone has different tolerances. On days when some people are wearing thick wetsuits, others are in their swim trunks with a rash guard.

Generally, there are three seasons of water temperatures. I have three different weight wetsuits because I am in the water all year. For the winter, I have a thick full wetsuit with a thickness called 4/3. This means the chest and back area have a layer that is 4 mm and the arms and legs have a layer that is 3 mm. The thicker layer keeps the core organs warmer.

This wetsuit is great for the winter when water temperatures in Oceanside drop into the 50's. More important for me because I am standing when I teach is resilience to the ocean breezes. For me, they are what make me get cold when I am in the water a few hours.

In the spring and fall when water temperatures are a little warmer, I have a full wetsuit that is the 3/2 thickness. In the summer when the water temperatures are above 70, I have a summer suit that has short sleeved arms and legs.

Wetsuits come in various qualities. My winter suit has a graphene lining which I find is terrific for both cold and wind. In general terms, a full 4/3 winter wet suit can run from $160 to $500. Depending on your country and water temperatures, different qualities may be necessary.

Sizes vary greatly. Each manufacturer has a chart on their website and they are based on weight and height. In my last research, wetsuits seem to top out at 3xxx large which is suitable up to 260 pounds. If you are larger, you might have to do more research to find a wetsuit.

Chapter Nineteen

Surf Training Can Change Your Lifestyle

When beginning on a venture it is good to have a worthwhile goal. A person beginning a nutrition and exercise program would be more motivated when he has an ambitious goal. He knows the challenge it will create and how fit he will have to be in order to be successful.

Navy Seals face some of the most rigorous training possible, but they know passing the tests are necessary to become a Seal. Only a few percent of the best qualified military personnel can pass the test. That alone is a badge of honor.

They are training to face the unknown. They may be training to accomplish extremely difficult or impossible missions. They may be facing another country's best military personnel or overwhelming obstacles. Landing in Pakistan a few miles from a military base to find Bin Laden was a daring task.

In face of these facts, learning to surf shouldn't be as difficult. It is not life threatening. In fact, it might be life-saving. Thinking of people accomplishing something more difficult than what you are trying to do might be encouragement that you can do it.

Everyone facing a challenge needs a good goal, discipline, focus, and resilience. In his book, "Resilience", Navy Seal and Rhodes scholar Eric Greitens said Seal Training is the greatest experience you never want to repeat. You learn how to face challenges you're not sure you can accomplish. What could be more fun than that?

One can wonder what goes through the mind of people like Elon Musk who keep doing what others would think is impossible. He took on the automotive industry with an electric car. He took on NASA by developing his own rocket ships. He built batteries big enough to bolster Australia's electric grid. Doesn't he ever worry about failure? Of course, he does.

One of the elements of surfing, I tell my students, is that fear is the 800-pound gorilla in the room. Most people have a little fear of the ocean's power. A wave is about speed and weight. It can weigh thousands of pounds when it falls on you if it is a big wave. One learns quickly that the power of waves is greater than a person's ability to withstand them without technique.

Champion big wave surfers said they were afraid each time they started surfing the next bigger sized waves. On real big days at Teahupoo, a big wave in Tahiti, recently, the surfers said they were even terrified, but this was their profession and what they chose in life.

A challenge might not be worthwhile if it doesn't scare you a little bit. It might not be worth your best efforts if there isn't a chance of failure. Doing what we know we can do is often boring. Doing work that is not challenging is stifling. Not growing is not your purpose.

The brain needs challenge to stay vital. Without challenge, it begins to decline. The end point of a declining brain is dementia. Its just a matter of time. We can learn all our lives because our brains have plasticity. Whenever you focus on something difficult that is a challenge, your brain grows. It is important to keep your brain growing.

If you are going to get healthy and fit so you can learn to surf, you are going to have lots of challenges. You are going to have to learn how to overcome obstacles. The biggest obstacle will be fighting your own willpower. You will have to make changes your mind will tell you are not good for you, at first.

The beauty of progressing is that soon your mind signs on to the mission and is your greatest fan. Exercise can become addicting. Someone starts off jogging, or weightlifting, or getting thinner and pretty soon they are addicted. The brain loves health and fitness.

Let's get started!

Source:

Chart for calculating the right volume surfboard for your weight.

From Website https://surfersfootprint.com/surfing-weight-limits-how-heavy-can-you-be-and-still-surf/

From the brand *Lost Boards*

Weight Range		Advanced	Inter/Advan	Intermediate	Inter/Beg	Beginner
LBS	KG		5% increase	25% increase	50% increase	100% increase
80	36.2	15.95	16.74	19.93	23.92	31.89
85	38.5	16.58	17.40	20.72	24.86	33.15
90	40.8	17.14	18.00	21.43	25.71	34.28
95	43.1	17.66	18.55	22.08	26.50	35.33
100	45.4	18.14	19.05	22.68	27.21	36.28
110	49.9	19.46	20.43	24.32	29.18	38.91
120	54.4	20.68	21.71	25.85	31.02	41.36
130	59.0	21.22	22.28	26.53	31.84	42.45
140	63.5	22.22	23.33	27.78	33.33	44.44
145	65.8	23.02	24.17	28.77	34.52	46.03
150	68.0	23.81	25.00	29.76	35.71	47.62
155	70.3	24.60	25.83	30.75	36.90	49.20
160	72.6	25.40	26.67	31.75	38.09	50.79
165	74.8	26.19	27.50	32.74	39.28	52.38
170	77.1	26.98	28.33	33.73	40.47	53.97
175	79.4	27.78	29.17	34.72	41.67	55.55
180	81.6	28.57	30.00	35.71	42.86	57.14
185	83.9	29.36	30.83	36.71	44.05	58.73
190	86.2	30.16	31.67	37.70	45.24	60.32
195	88.4	30.95	32.50	38.69	46.43	61.90
200	90.7	31.75	33.33	39.68	47.62	63.49
210	95.2	33.33	35.00	41.67	50.00	66.66
220	99.8	35.92	37.71	44.90	53.88	71.83
230	104.3	38.59	40.52	48.24	57.89	77.19
240	108.8	41.36	43.43	51.70	62.04	82.72

Bibliography

Mark Kaplan

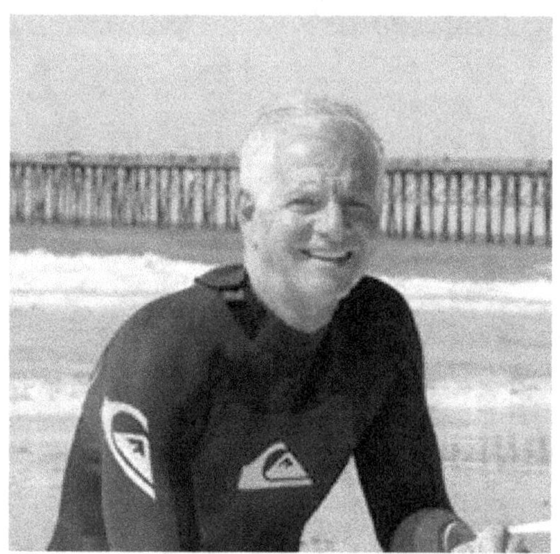

I have been a life-long enthusiast of exercise and health. Most sports and recreation have been attractive to me and I have tried as many as possible. My love was running and I started jogging in high school and running more seriously with a community track club as an adult.

Surfing was a high school adventure but became more of an addiction after I retired. Daily surfing and website building for others led to a surfing website which became highly rated by Google for surf lessons in Oceanside. This became my accidental backing into the business of teaching surf lessons.

Noticing how many of my students from kids to seniors were overweight and not in good condition led me to a certification by Ace as a Health Coach. I also pursued courses in Personal Training and Nutrition.

Surfing is just one great goal for motivating a change in one's personal fitness. Pursuing health and fitness is a lifestyle and affords many benefits. I hope this book leads to your desire to make lifestyle changes.